Dash Diet Weight Loss Solution

Dash Diet for Beginners, Action Plan for Weight Loss

Olivia White

Legal & Disclaimer

The information contained in this book and its contents is not designed to replace or take the place of any form of medical or professional advice; and is not meant to replace the need for independent medical, financial, legal or other professional advice or services, as may be required. The content and information in this book has been provided for educational and entertainment purposes only.

The content and information contained in this book has been compiled from sources deemed reliable, and it is accurate to the best of the Author's knowledge, information and belief. However, the Author cannot guarantee its accuracy and validity and cannot be held liable for any errors and/or omissions. Further, changes are periodically made to this book as and when needed. Where appropriate and/or necessary, you must consult a professional (including but not limited to your doctor, attorney, financial advisor or such other professional advisor) before using any of the suggested remedies, techniques, or information in this book.

Upon using the contents and information contained in this book, you agree to hold harmless the Author from and against any damages, costs, and expenses, including any legal fees potentially resulting from the application of any of the information provided by this book. This disclaimer applies to any loss, damages or injury caused by the use and application, whether directly or indirectly, of any advice or information presented, whether for breach of contract, tort, negligence, personal injury, criminal intent, or under any other cause of action.

You agree to accept all risks of using the information presented inside this book.

You agree that by continuing to read this book, where appropriate and/or necessary, you shall consult a professional (including but not limited to your doctor, attorney, or financial advisor or such other advisor as needed) before using any of the suggested remedies, techniques, or information in this book.

Introduction

The book you are going to read may not give you all information about diets, but it will explain to you how healthy food could improve the quality of your life. It will also change your attitude to your health and show you how tasty healthy meals could be.

Nowadays, so many people around the world suffer from different diseases. But so often they just forget that such problems come from the bad eating habits which have an awful influence on their health. Because usually we even don't understand how big is the role of nutrition in the life. Not everyone even thinks about the importance of healthy meals for the health. But, actually, what we eat plays one of the main roles in how we feel day by day.

This book will tell you about a healthy diet, keeping on which will improve your health as well as your life. The DASH diet is recommended according to the many types of research. It is known as absolutely safe and healthy way for reducing high blood pressure (or preventing it) and losing weight. Moreover, it is a best-selling diet, which is very helpful as a healthy diet against different diseases and illnesses. It includes the dietary plan, following which will help you to solve your health problems without making any stress for your body.

This diet has already helped millions of people all around the world to lower the blood pressure, to lose extra weight or just to improve their health. So if you have any of these problems, be sure that this book will be your personal beneficial guide on the way to the better and healthier life. It will teach you everything that you need to know about healthy and tasty food.

Table of Contents

1.Dash diet basics

Thanks to the nowadays researchers, there are different safe ways which are very helpful for improving your health, especially if you have some serious problems with it. One of such method is the DASH diet (Dietary Approaches to Stop Hypertension). It is also known as an example of diet, which was recommended by USA National Institute of Heart, Lungs, and Blood.

The main purpose of this diet is to prevent and control high blood pressure (hypertension – medical term). The DASH diet helps you to reduce the sodium in your daily ration and eat different food full of nutrients (potassium, magnesium, calcium) which are very helpful in making your blood pressure lower. Choosing such diet, your blood pressure can be reduced by a few points just in three weeks. After some time, you will see, that your blood pressure lower by eight-twelve points, that can greatly reduce the risk of serious diseases. Following the DASH diet guarantees you to make your eating habits healthier. It will not only lower your blood pressure but also it offers health benefits. Furthermore, this diet is recommended by nutritionists for preventing such diseases as cancer, osteoporosis, stroke, diabetes and other heart illnesses. The DASH diet is very rich in vegetables, fruits, whole grains and, of course, low-fat dairy products (organic soy milk or almond milk etc.) This diet also includes such products as fish, meat, beans, and nuts. Everything sweet (chocolate, cookies or cakes), drinks full of sugar, as well as red meat and products with extra fat should be limited during this diet. The DASH diet can be considered as a great example of diet for any social groups, not only for those people, who suffer from high blood pressure. Also, this diet is very well-balanced, that is why it has a great effect on cholesterol level and water retention in your body.

One of the main advantages of this diet that there is no need to be or to become a professional chef. You don't have to spend hours in your kitchen, reading lots of cooking books. Healthy food is very easy and quick to cook. All you need is just to analyze what you eat normally. As soon as you have done it, try to correct your daily ration. Of course, it may be not so easy to do, but if you want to start it, don't let yourself to put it off. Just start it from this moment and be sure after two weeks or even less you'll feel absolutely differently than now. Don't worry, this diet will teach you how to choose healthy food and how to make delicious dishes from it.

The problem with blood pressure can touch everyone. The higher it is the more risk it can make for your health. Studies have shown that the level of the blood pressure directly depends on what people eat. Besides all healthy food that the DASH diet includes, it also focuses on the amount of sodium that we eat. Because too much salt in food increases the level of the blood pressure. That is why the DASH diet also provides you with some recommendations about how to intake less salt.

The optimal amount of the salt for person per day is not more than 1 tsp (=7 grams). But it's a norm only for those who don't have any chronic diseases (especially heart diseases!) The recommended amount of the salt for people suffering from hypertension, diabetes (second type), chronic kidney diseases and also for people who are older than 51 years, is only 3-4 grams per day. But you should understand that this daily amount includes all salt that we eat during the day, not only pure salt but also so-called "hidden" from other products. Such products that contain this "hidden" salt are all possible canned goods, ready-to-cook food, all sorts of sausages, meat and fish smoked products, chips, popcorn, marinades, fast food, salted nuts, ketchup and many different sauces. This list can be easily added because sometimes we even can imagine how much salt we eat for sure.

However, if you want to stay healthy, it is better to refuse from eating such food. You won't lose anything except some plus kilograms. Actually, it is much easier to stop eating all these products, than to control every gram of the salt you eat. Here are some tips, following which will help you to reduce the salt intake:

1. Don't salt food while cooking. Especially, if you are cooking for your family. Let everyone to salt food himself. It can be a problem only for the first couple of the days.
2. Instead of salt, use herbs, spices or lemon juice.
3. Instead of buying canned goods, buy fresh food and cook whatever you like.
4. Don't take frozen ready-to-cook food (pizza, nuggets and so on). They usually have a lot of salt.
5. Instead of different sausages, it's better to eat real meat.
6. Eat more fresh vegetables and fruits. Even if you buy some frozen vegetables or fruits (during the winter time, for example) try to find with "no-salt-added"
7. To reduce the amount of salt in such products as tuna, rinse it.
8. Limit in your ration such food as bacon, ham, pickled vegetables, soy sauce and teriyaki etc.
9. Limit such seasoning as mustard, pickles and many other sauces that contain salt ingredients.
10. While buying food, pay attention to food labels. It will help you to compare the amount of salt in products and to choose food which is lower in salt and total fat.

Another important thing before starting the DASH dietary program is your medication (for controlling blood pressure) If you take such tablets, don't stop it. Consult with your doctor about your treatment and start to follow the DASH diet.

Even for those who don't have problems with blood pressure, the DASH diet plan will be helpful for losing extra weight or for controlling your blood pressure on the normal level. Try to combine your diet plan with some kind of physical activities, such as running, swimming or just walking. Such activity will take only twenty or thirty minutes every day. But if you are very busy and don't have enough time for sport, try to start walking every morning and evening for fifteen minutes.

To be more motivated, make a special physical activity program for yourself: set new goals for every day to maintain interest. The important thing is to do everything with pleasure and to do only what you really like. If you don't want to give up very fast, don't try to do your maximum from the start. Moreover, if you have some chronic heart problem, consult with your doctor before starting any physical activity program.

Try to compare what is on your plate with your dietary program, this will show what changes should be done in your usual food choices. First of all, to start your DASH dietary program you have to focus on the main principles of it, following which will give you the better result.

1. The calorific value shouldn't be bigger than 2000 – 2500 kcal per day.
2. Daily salt intake should be lowered, especially for hypertensive patients.
3. It is also necessary to avoid drinking alcohol and cigarettes.
4. Limit the amount of fat and salt in your ration. Replace your favorite products with low-fat or fat-free analogs.
5. Instead of chocolate, cakes and everything sweet, try to eat more vegetables and fruits, which are full of vitamins.
6. Include in your daily meal low-fat dairy products, beans, nuts and whole wheat bread.
7. It's better to eat more products, which are rich in magnesium, calcium, and potassium.

Don't forget that any kind of diet shouldn't be stressful for your body. Try to follow it step by step and don't make a quick jump because then you won't have an expected result. Too fast losing weight is bad for your health and may cause other problems. The purpose of the DASH diet isn't just to make you slim, the purpose of this diet is to improve your health by changing your eating habits and teaching you how to make your lifestyle healthier than it is. The DASH dietary program can be started with replacing some products from your usual ration. With the help of these tips, you will find it easier to start the DASH diet:

1. Every time you have a lunch or a dinner, add some vegetables to your meal.

2. Make a dessert from fruits or eat them like a snack. Be sure, you'll enjoy it. Also, you can find a lot of different recipes in the cooking book or on the internet (cooking blogs will help you). Believe that some fresh fruits canned in their own juice can be very tasty.

3. If you like dairy products, try to replace them with the low-fat (1-2 %) or even fat-free (skim) products. But if you don't like such dairy products, try to drink something lactose-free or almond milk. It will also help you to reduce your daily intake of fat, cholesterol and the total amount of calories.

4. Instead of eating junk snacks such as chips with different tastes, try to make a mix of nuts or resins; buy fat-free or low-fat yogurts or frozen yogurt instead of your favorite chocolate ice-cream. If you are a popcorn fan, buy it without butter and salt added.

5. While choosing food, read carefully what is written on the labels. Avoid buying products which include a big amount of sodium.

6. If it is hard for you to make your portion smaller, add more vegetables to your meal. In this case, you don't need to change the dish size.

7. Also, don't forget that meat is just a part of your dish. It shouldn't be the main ingredient on your plate That is why it is better to eat low-fat meat. If it is possible, 2-3 meals per weak should be without meat. Then choose 2-3 days per week for being a little bit vegetarian. Don't forget that meat can be replaced by mushrooms or fish.

All these tips will give you a great support on the beginning of your dietary program. For making these process more successful, take a new diary where you will write small notes about your little achievements. A few days later try to read your notes again: it will help you to see the whole picture of how your eating habits are changing. You will also see what should be corrected. Maybe you have a bad habit to miss your breakfast and then have small snacks, eating something sweet or even salty. Use this dairy at least for one week. It will allow you to understand yourself as well as all your eating habits better. It also will identify even small problems which require immediate solutions from your side.

The DASH diet is a very helpful dietary program for those who want to lose their weight but don't know how to do this in a good healthy way. If you still don't believe that it works without any bad effects on your health, the ten reasons you are going to read will make you believe in this diet.

1. Being on the DASH won't make you feel hungry. There is no need to drink only water and to forget about food. Healthy meal and workout will give you a great result in losing your extra weight.

2. As soon as you have started the DASH dietary program, day by day you would realize, that you get used to eating normal healthy food. And just believe, you will easily forget what the taste of fast food and coca cola is.

3. Following this dietary program won't be harmful to your budget. You don't need to pay an enormous amount of the money to eat healthy food.
4. Of course, cooking healthy food takes time, but it also gives you a possibility to learn what is good for your health. The DASH diet will teach you how to choose healthy eating for the rest of your life.
5. Eating more vegetables and fruits will help you to lose weight faster. Because fruits and vegetables contain fiber which speeds up your metabolism.
6. The DASH dietary program includes only healthy food. And as you know many nutritional factors influence not only your blood pressure but also your weight.
7. In combination with calorie reduction and sport, it gives you a possibility to become more fit and to have a body of your dream.
8. Of course, the weight loss isn't so effortless and easy, as most of the people want it to be, but keeping on the DASH dietary program will make losing weight simple. One of the main purposes of this program is to show you how to calculate calories you should eat every day.
9. This program won't let you overeat. Because at the minimum, according to the DASH diet, you have to eat three meals a day. That is why you have no chance to skip the meal.
10. There is no need to leave your plate clean every time. It's better to eat until you will feel 70 or 80 percent full. Taking fruits or nuts as a small snack would be rather better for you.

For those, who want to lose weight, the DASH diet includes as much healthy food as you need for losing weight. You just have to move more and eat less. But you have to remember that the DASH diet isn't a magic weight-loss solution. Yes, eating healthier food might help you to lose weight, but for the more effective result, you should include sport in your plan. That is the simple secret of how to be healthy and beautiful. If you will follow all these recommendations as well as the DASH dietary program, you will feel better very soon.

Following such dietary program will demonstrate you, how to make it a part of your new lifestyle, of your healthy lifestyle. Even if you slip from your diet for a few days, don't be afraid, it is quite normal for all people to slip when they try something new. On the way to reaching your health goals don't forget that this process needs your time as well as your patience but be sure that you can change everything you want, especially what is on your plate.

2. Losing weight on the DASH diet

It is known that the DASH diet was developed not only for losing extra weight but for lowering blood pressure. However, according to its dietary program, it is rich in low-calorie products. You can easily replace some of them with healthy food, which has fewer calories but more benefits for your health. That is why eating healthier food will also help you to lose your weight.

The benefit of the DASH diet is confirmed by scientists as well as by people who have tried this kind of diet. It was proved, that a special effect can be achieved if you combine diet with physical exercises. Medical research has shown that in four weeks being on the DASH diet helps to lose eight or even ten kilograms, of course, it depends on your weight. Moreover, without physical exercises weight loss will be smaller. And according to some studies, those adults who went on the DASH diet lost more weight than those who tried other low-calorie diets. It proves that this kind of the diet may help you not only to lose some weight but also make you healthier (what, actually, many other diets don't do). At the same time, you have to realize that the effect of losing weight from the DASH diet isn't extremely fast, but it is stable and natural. Losing weight in such way won't interrupt or break the normal function of the body.

So if you have any problems with your weight, try to combine your healthy diet with the sport. As it was mentioned before, it can be anything you like to do: walking before going to bed, running every morning (you don't have to be a professional running, make it easy – just start from 15-20 minutes every morning), swimming, playing any sport games (especially, if you have kids) or just morning exercising with music etc. Even if you aren't an athletic person, try to start from something small, doing it day by day, soon you will see how your body become more fit.

Before starting your personal sports career, make a schedule for every day and try to keep it. It will help you to plan your day in a smart way and to find time for everything that you need or want. Then, if you are afraid to give up very fast, ask your friend or family member to join you. Let somebody have a chance to be more fit too. But, if seriously, somebody can just keep you motivated. At the same time, you will be a support for each other. Another component is the activity you choose: try to mix it with something new, for example, running with swimming. Different activities have a better effect on the body.

As in any process, set goals. Even every small achievement should be celebrated. Your mood is very significant it will give you good energy to carry on. So don't be shy to be proud of yourself, don't wait when somebody will make you a compliment. That will teach you how to self-motivated person.

Another visible thing that should be mentioned is the aim of your DASH dietary program. To make it correctly, according to the DASH diet rules, you have to consider the goal – health recovery or just weight loss. So if you want to lose weight, you will have to make a diet for yourself (better with a help of a specialist in this question). Because the purpose of the DASH diet isn't just to control an amount of food, but also to control the quality of food that you eat daily. And be sure, that it is an absolutely flexible eating plan which won't make you stay or even feel hungry.

The DASH dietary program can be made based on the general diet rules, which count your healthy food in the right portions.

The daily ration of the DASH diet can be formed, based on such (helpful) rules:
1. Don't forget to drink about 2 liters of the mineral water per day.
2. 5 fruits: one portion – one fruit or ½ glass of juice.
3. 5 different vegetables.
4. Beans and nuts: 5 portions per week or 40 grams per day.
5. One or two spoons of olive oil, which can be added to the salad, for example.

6. The necessary dose of protein should be about 200 grams of lean meat, fish or eggs per day.
7. Not more than 3 portions of the law-far dairy products.
8. Very important is to reduce the amount of sugar (as well as salt) in your ration. Try to eat honey instead of sugar, but not more than 1 tsp.

There is a huge variety of products which you can eat during the DASH diet. They are not only healthy but tasty too. Of course, you have to remember about the serving sizes of what you eat even if this food is good for your health.

The list below will tell you all healthy food that the DASH diet offers. It also will illustrate the benefit of each product.

- Whole grains which contain a lot of minerals and nutrients. Adding them to your meal will help you to reduce the risk of high blood pressure.
- Fruits. A lot of fruits are rich in potassium (bananas, for example) which maintains fluid in our body. Also, it is known as a great heart helper. And the surprising fact that was proved by studies is that eating 2 bananas per day for more than one week can lower your blood pressure by 10-12 %. But if you don't like bananas, you can find potassium in oranges, lemons, grapefruits or avocados. Other good protectors against the high blood pressure are blueberries, strawberries, raspberries, black currants etc.
- Vegetables. They are known as a wonderful source of fiber and other useful vitamins and minerals. If you still have no idea how to add more vegetables and fruits to your typical menu, the American Heart Association has invented a special chart, which organizes them by color (you can easily with it online)
- Dairy products. All we know that such products are rich in calcium and protein. It can be a surprise but low-fat dairy products or even fat-free have magnesium and potassium, which are good for your heart.
- Of course, don't forget about lean meat and fish. Meat is very reached in vitamins B, iron, magnesium, vitamin E, zinc, and protein. Actually, it is the biggest resource of protein. And as about fish, it has a high level of omega-3 fatty acids. Omega-3 lower the risk or the different heart diseases, stroke, heart attack or even death.
- Nuts and seeds. Nuts also contain a lot of protein and "good" fats which reduce bad cholesterol level.

This list can be added endless. Because the benefit of healthy food is bigger than you can imagine. But even eating healthy food you shouldn't forget that everything should have reasonable limits. That is why, while following this diet, try to pay your attention to the serving sizes. Of course, it doesn't mean that you have to stay hungry, but in any case, it is better to eat a little bit less than to overeat every time.

Also, there are some daily nutritional recommendations according to the DASH dietary program. Such example may help you to form your eating plan and to choose better products with more benefits for your health. Furthermore, it will show you how to calculate the calories in a proper way.

- Carbohydrates should be not more than 55 % of your daily calories.
- Good cholesterol should be limited to 150 mg per day.
- As for the protein – only 18 % of all calories.
- The daily norm of fiber is 30 grams. Better if more.
- Total fat shouldn't be more than 25 % of the daily calories.
- As for saturated fat – only 5 % or even less.

Moreover, before going on the DASH diet, you have to choose which one is suitable for you. There are forms of the DASH diet: the standard DASH diet – where sodium should be limited to 2, 300 mg per day; the lower-sodium DASH diet – where sodium consumption should be not more than 1, 500 mg per day. Depending on your health needs, you have to make a choice which one is good for you. But if you aren't sure, it is better to consult with the doctor. So here are some recommended daily food servings according to the DASH diet (for 2000 calories per day):

- Fruits – 4-5 a day (one serving is one medium size fruit or 200 ml of fresh juice)
- Vegetables 5-6 a day (one serving ½ cup cooking vegetables such as carrots, broccoli, mushrooms, corn, potatoes or green beans)
- Grains – 7-8 a day (one serving is one slice of bread or ½ cup of rice, pasta)
- Low-fat or fat-free dairy products – 2 (where 1 portion = 1 glass of milk or yogurt)
- Nuts – 4-5 portions per week (where 1 portion = 1/3 cup)
- Fats and oils – 2-3 portions per day (1 portion = 1 tsp margarine, 1 tsp olive oil or 2 tsp of salad dressing)
- Lean meat or fish – 200 gr of cooked lean meat.
- Sweets and sugar – 5 or even less per week (1 portion = 1 tbsp of sugar). But it will be much better instead of sugar use honey (only natural!)
- Sodium: 2, 300 mg per day. Or 1, 500 mg – if you have any health problems.
- Alcohol. Only 1-2 drinks per day. For women, the maximum is 1 drink per day (150 ml of wine), for men it can be 2 drinks per day but not more.

There is no single diet plan. Depending on your personal health or weight loss needs, you can choose another DASH diet plan that provides different number of calories (from 1, 200 to 3, 100 calories per day)

Such list is just an example of what size servings should be. But you have to realize that serving size depends on the number of calories which you eat daily. Knowing the serving size will let you make your own meal plan for the whole day or even for the whole week. With the help of such plan, you will not only become healthier but you will also improve your life.

3. Your first 28 days

As everything new, going on diet is very hard. Firstly, because keeping on the healthy diet means that you have to change your eating habits, especially if they are unhealthy. The second and, actually, the biggest problem is that you should leave your usual comfort zone because only desire to change something isn't enough. That is why, if you read this because you want to make your life better and, of course, healthier, you have to be honest, first of all, with yourself to see what and how should be changed in your daily meal. For that reason, this book offers you a kind of a dietary challenge, which will not only improve your health condition but will also change your attitude to the healthy food.

The 28 days DASH dietary program offers you to try the diet, following which will make you feel better, stronger and healthier. And be sure, in the end of this so-called little challenge, your eating habits will differ from those, that you used to have.

Here you will find an example of the DASH dietary plan for 28 days. This plan will include three meals for each day during the week plus some small snacks. Remember that for having the more effective result, you have to follow this plan strictly. You will also need time to prepare meals for yourself, so don't be lazy. Pay attention that the menu below is calculated for the ration of 2000 calories per day. Moreover, all meal plans correspond to the recommended intake of vitamins and minerals for people who are older than 50. Also, you can replace some food with products that you like, but only if they are from one category. For example, while replacing vegetables or fruits, try to find alternative variants, which are rich in potassium. Furthermore, try to choose lean meat, fish, and low-fat or even fat-free dairy products.

First week

Day 1. Monday
Breakfast: corn flakes with a toast and a glass of juice.
- 30 g corn flakes with 180 grams of blueberries
- 180 ml orange juice (or apple juice)
- 1 whole-grain toast with 2 tsp. strawberry jam
- 230 ml low-fat milk

Lunch: chicken sandwich and a green salad.
- Small sandwich with chicken breast
- Salad: lettuce, 9 cherry tomatoes. 2 tbsp. low-fat dressing
- 230 ml milk
- 1 medium apple (or orange)

Snack: fresh yogurt with nuts.
- ¼ cup almonds
- 180 ml raspberry yogurt (sugar-free)

Dinner: chicken chop with potatoes, green salad, green beans, cookies, and grapes.
- 180 g chicken chop
- ½ cup of green beans
- Green salad with 2 tbsp. of olive oil and vinegar
- 2-3 cookies
- 1 glass of grapes

Daily portions:
- 3 servings whole grains
- 4 fruits
- 5 vegetables
- 3 serving low-fat dairy products
- 40 g nuts
- 200 g meat

Day 2. Tuesday
Breakfast: Omelet, toast, juice, berries, and latte.
- 2 whole-grain toast with 4 tsp. strawberry jam (or blueberry)
- 1 cup different fresh berries: strawberries, raspberries, and blueberries
- 180 ml orange juice
- Latte: 240 ml of low-fat milk

Lunch: Ham, sandwich, fresh vegetables, and apple.
- Sandwich: 2 pieces whole-grain bread 60 g ham, 30 g low-fat cheese, ¼ cup of shredded cabbage, 2 slices tomato and mustard
- ½ cup fresh carrot
- 8 cherry tomatoes
- 1 medium apple (or orange)

Snack: Hazelnut, melon, and yogurt.
- ¼ cup hazelnut
- 120 g melon
- 180 g low-fat kiwi (peach) yogurt

Dinner: Salmon with mashed potatoes, broccoli, salad, bread and frozen yogurt (instead of ice-cream)

- 120 g grilled salmon
- ½ cup mashed potatoes
- 1 cup steamed broccoli
- ½ cup vegetables with 2 tbsp. of dressing
- 1 piece of bread
- ½ cup low-fat frozen yogurt (sugar-free)

Daily servings:

- 4 servings of green-grain products
- 3 servings of low-fat dairy products
- 4 fruits
- 5 (+/-) vegetables
- 40 g of nuts
- 240 g of meat

Day 3. Wednesday

Breakfast: Tasty French toast with fruits and a fresh smoothie.

- 2 whole-grain toast with the ½ cup of sliced peaches (or strawberries)
- Smoothie: 120 g of strawberries, ½ banana and 240 ml low-fat milk

Lunch: Sandwich with tuna and cheese, potatoes, cabbage salad, milk and some fruits.

- Sandwich: ½ cup of tuna, 30 g of low-fat cheese and 1 piece of whole-grain bread
- 1 serving of baked potatoes
- 1 serving of cabbage salad
- ½ cup steamed peas and carrots
- 240 ml low-fat milk
- 1 medium apple (or banana)

Afternoon snack. Fresh carrots, cheese, almond.

- 8 small fresh carrots with low-fat cheese
- ¼ cup of almond

Dinner: Grilled chicken with young vegetables, baked potatoes, spinach, some berries, and plums.

- Grilled chicken
- ½ cup young vegetables and 4 tomatoes with 2 tbsp. dressing
- ½ cup baked potatoes
- ½ cup spinach
- 1 cup of berries and 2 plumps

Daily servings:

- 3 servings of whole grains
- 4 fruits
- 5-6 vegetables
- 3 servings of dairy products
- 40 g nuts
- 180 g meat

Day 4. Thursday
Breakfast: Omelet, strawberries, toast, juice, and milk.
- Omelet: ½ cup milk-egg mixture
- 180 g sliced strawberries
- 1 whole-grain toast with 2 tsp strawberry (blueberry) jam
- 180 ml orange juice
- 240 ml low-fat milk

Lunch: Sandwich with beef and cheese, potato chips (home-made) with tomatoes, a glass of milk, and some fruits.
- Sandwich: 2 pieces of whole-grain bread, 60 g lean meat, 30 g low-fat cheese, ¼ cup lettuce, 2 slices of tomato, and mustard (or without it)
- 30 g low-salted potato chips cooked in the oven
- 4 tomatoes
- 230 ml low-fat milk
- 2 peaches

Afternoon snack: Apple slices and low-fat yogurt.
- 1 medium sliced apple
- 1 low-fat yogurt

Dinner: Spaghetti with low-fat sauce, green beans, lettuce and frozen yogurt for a dessert.
- Spaghetti with the low-fat sauce: 1 cup sauce and 1 cup spaghetti
- ½ cup of green beans
- Green salad: ½ cup lettuce with 2 tbsp. low-fat Italian sauce, without salt
- ½ cup of frozen yogurt (sugar-free)

Servings:
- 3 servings of whole-grain bread
- 4 fruits
- 5 vegetables
- 4 (+/-) servings of low-fat dairy products
- 40 g of nuts
- 200 g of meat

Day 5. Friday
Breakfast: Small muffins (or cookies) with yogurt. Fresh juice and low-fat milk.
- 2 small muffins (or three small cookies)
- 180 ml of low-fat kiwi (or peach) yogurt
- 180 ml of orange (or apple) juice
- 240 ml of low-fat milk

Lunch: Roll with turkey, cheese, and cranberries, salad, peach.
- Roll: whole-grain bread, ¼ cup of cranberry sauce, 90 g of turkey breast, 30 g of low-fat cheese
- Salad: 1 cup of vegetables with 1 tbsp. of olive oil and vinegar
- 1 medium peach

Snack: Yogurt, walnuts and some berries.
- 150 ml of low-fat yogurt
- 40 g of walnuts
- ½ cup of different berries

Dinner: Pork chop with baked potatoes, sauce, tomatoes and lettuce.
- 150 g lean pork chop
- 1 cup of baked potatoes
- ¼ cup of low-fat sauce
- Salad: ½ cup of vegetables, 3 tomatoes and 2 tbsp. of French dressing

Servings:
- 1 serving of whole-grain products
- 4 fruits
- 6 (+/-) vegetables
- 3 (+/-) servings of low-fat dairy products
- 40 g of nuts
- 240 g of meat

Day 6. Saturday

Breakfast: English muffin with cheese, melon, juice, and milk.
- 1 muffin with cinnamon and raisins with low-fat cheese
- 180 g of melon
- 180 ml of orange juice
- 240 ml of low-fat milk

Lunch: Pork tacos with peach
- 90 g of lean meat for tacos
- 30 g of low-fat cheese
- Sliced tomatoes and romaine salad, grated carrots, and chopped red cabbage
- 1 medium peach

Snack: Apple, popcorn, cheese.
- 1 medium apple
- 2 cups of popcorn
- 1 piece of low-fat cheese

Dinner: Steak, baked potatoes, broccoli, lettuce.
- 120 g of beef steak
- 1 baked potato
- ½ cup of broccoli
- Salad: 1 ½ of leafy vegetables with 2 tbsp. of sauce
- 1 piece of whole-grain bread with 1 tsp. of soft margarine
- 180 ml of low-fat peach yogurt (sugar-free)

Daily servings:
- 5 servings of whole-grain products
- 4 fruits
- 5 vegetables
- 3 (+/-) servings of dairy products
- 40 g of nuts
- 210 g of meat

Day 7. Sunday

Breakfast: Omelet with cheese, cookies, milk, and juice.
- Omelet with low-fat cheese

- 180 ml of orange juice
- 240 ml of low-fat milk
- 2 cookies

Lunch: Cheese with tomato, cucumber salad, and peaches.

- 2 pieces of whole-grain bread, 20 g of low-fat cheese and 2 tomato slices
- ¾ cup of cucumber slices and 1 tbsp. of low-fat Italian dressing.
- 1 peach

Snack: Yogurt, peanuts, and melon.

- 180 ml of low-fat strawberry yogurt.
- ¼ cup of roasted peanut (without salt)
- 180 g of melon

Dinner: Grilled chicken with potatoes, vegetables, pudding and some fruits.

- 1 serving of grilled chicken with potatoes, carrots, Brussel sprouts
- ½ cup of chocolate pudding
- 1 medium pear

Servings:

- 2 servings of whole-grain products
- 5 fruits
- 5 (+/-) vegetables
- 3 (+/-) servings of dairy products
- 40 g of nuts
- 240 g of lean meat

Second week

Breakfast: Scrambled eggs, toast, pineapple, juice and milk.

- 2 eggs
- 2 whole-grain toast and 4 tsp. orange marmalade
- 180 g pineapple
- 180 ml orange juice
- 240 ml low-fat milk

Lunch: Salad with chicken, whole-grain bread, Italian cabbage salad, milk, strawberries, jelly, and plums.

- ½ salad with chicken
- 1 whole-grain cake
- 1 cup of Italian cabbage salad
- 240 ml of low-fat milk
- ½ cup of strawberry jelly
- 1 medium plum

Snack: Yogurt with banana

- 180 ml of low-fat yogurt
- 1 medium banana

Dinner: Grilled chicken with potatoes, green salad, and frozen yogurt.

- Grilled chicken – 120 g
- 1 cup of potatoes
- 1 cup of asparagus
- Salad: 1 ½ cup of greens and vegetables, 2 tbsp. of olive oil and vinegar
- 1 cup of low-fat yogurt

Servings:

- 3 servings of the whole-grain products
- 4 (+/-) fruits
- 6 vegetables
- 4 servings of dairy products
- 240 g of meat

Breakfast: Muffin with peanut butter, orange, and milk.

- 1 muffin with 1 tbsp. of natural peanut butter
- 180ml of strawberry yogurt
- 1 medium orange
- 240 ml of low-fat milk

Lunch: Vegetable burger with baked potatoes, cabbage salad, and banana.

- Vegetable burger: grilled vegetable loaf, low-fat cheese, 2 slices of tomato, ¼ romaine lettuce
- 1 serving of baked potatoes
- ½ cup of cabbage salad
- 1 banana

Snack: Yogurt, pear, and walnuts.

- 180 ml of low-fat kiwi yogurt
- 1 pear
- 40 g of walnuts

Dinner: Grilled chicken breast with baked potatoes, carrots, green salad and frozen yogurt.
- 120 g of grilled chicken
- 1 baked potato
- 1 cup of fresh carrots
- Green salad: 1 ½ cup of different vegetables, 2 tbsp. of Italian dressing
- ½ cup of chocolate low-fat frozen yogurt

Servings:
- 4 serving of whole-grain products
- 3 fruits
- 6-7 vegetables
- 4 servings of dairy products
- 1 serving of beans
- 40 g of nuts
- 120 g of meat

Day 10. Wednesday

Breakfast: Oatmeal, banana, toast, grapefruit, and milk.
- ½ cup of oatmeal with small pieces of banana
- 1 whole-grain toast with 2 tsp. of orange jam
- 180 g of grapefruit
- 240 ml of low-fat milk

Lunch: Soup, cheese, yogurt, and apples.
- 1 cup of vegetable soup
- 30 g of low-fat cheese
- 180 ml of low-fat yogurt
- 2 small apples

Snack: Cheese and berries.
- 1 piece of low-fat cheese
- 1/3 cup of different fresh berries

Dinner: Pork chop with baked potatoes, green beans, carrot salad, walnuts, and milk.
- 120 g of fried pork chop
- ½ cup of baked potatoes
- 1 cup of green beans
- ½ cup of carrot salad with ¼ cup of nuts
- 240 ml of low-fat milk

Daily servings:
- 3 portions of whole-grain products
- 4 fruits
- 7 vegetables
- 4 (+/-) servings of dairy products
- 1 serving of nuts
- 120 g of meat

Breakfast: Cornflakes, melon, apple juice, milk.

- 45 g corn flakes
- 180 g melon
- 180 ml orange juice
- 240 ml low-fat milk

Lunch: Cheese, green salad, fresh vegetables, and orange.

- 2 pieces of whole-grain bread with 30 low-fat cheese and 2 slices of tomato
- Salad: 1 cup of vegetables with 2 tbsp. of French sauce
- 8 small carrots
- 1 medium orange

Snack: Strawberry smoothie with almonds

- Smoothie: 240 ml low-fat milk and 180 g strawberries
- 40 g almonds

Dinner: Grilled chicken with rice and broccoli. Cheese and lettuce.

- 1 serving of grilled chicken
- 1 cup white rice
- ½ cup broccoli with 30 g melted low-fat cheese
- Salad: 1 ½ cup of vegetables with 2 tbsp. of dressing

Daily servings:

- 3 servings of whole-grain products
- 1 serving of nuts
- 5 fruits
- 3 servings of dairy products
- 210 g of lean meat

Day 12. Friday

Breakfast: Cornflakes, banana, milk, and juice.

- 30 g cornflakes with small banana pieces
- 180 ml strawberry juice
- 240 ml milk

Lunch: Pita with tuna, salad, and grapes.

- Pita with tuna: ½ whole-grain pita with ½ cup of tuna and with 2 slices of tomato
- Salad: 1 cup of leafy vegetables with 2 tbsp. of dressing
- 180 g grapes

Snack: Peanuts with plums

- ¼ cup of peanuts
- 2 plums

Dinner: Cheeseburger with cabbage salad, and ice-cream.

- Low-fat cheeseburger: 120 g of low-fat beef, 30 g of low-fat cheese, 2 tomato slices, lettuce and bread for burger
- ½ cabbage salad
- 1 cup broccoli and carrots
- Ice-cream: 30 g of raspberries with low-fat frozen yogurt

Daily servings:

- 2 servings of whole-grain products

- 4 fruits
- 5 vegetables
- 3 servings of dairy products
- 40 g nuts
- 210 g meat

Day 13. Saturday

Breakfast: Bagel with cheese, some fruits, hot chocolate, and juice.
- ½ of whole-grain bagel with low-fat cheese
- 180 g strawberries
- 240 ml hot chocolate: 240 ml low-fat milk with 1 tsp. cocoa
- 180 ml orange juice

Lunch: Burrito with cheese and beans, lettuce, and apples.
- 1 burrito with ½ cup beans and 20 g low-fat cheese
- ½ cup corn
- Salad: 1 cup lettuce, tomatoes, and carrots with 1 tbsp. nuts and 1 tbsp. olive oil
- 2 small apples

Snack: Latte, cookies, fruit salad.
- Coffee Latte
- 2 biscuits
- ½ cup fruit salad

Dinner: Steak with salad, fruit chips.
- 120 g steak
- Green salad: 1 ½ cup vegetables with 2 tbsp. olive oil and vinegar
- ½ cup fruit crisps with ½ cup low-fat frozen yogurt

Servings:
- 3 servings of whole-grain products
- 5 fruits
- 5 vegetables
- 5 serving of low-fat dairy products
- 40 g beans
- 120 g meat

Day 14. Sunday

Breakfast: Scrambled eggs, pineapple, juice, milk.
- Scrambled eggs with 3 slices of avocado
- 180 g pineapple
- 180 g apple juice
- 240 ml low-fat milk for latte

Lunch: Spaghetti Bolognese, salad, juice, and berries.
- 150 g spaghetti Bolognese
- Salad: 1 cup fresh vegetables with 2 tbsp. olive oil
- 180 ml orange juice
- 1/3 cup berries

Snack: Tomato soup, orange.
- ¾ cup tomato soup

- 1 medium orange

Dinner: Rice with vegetables and frozen yogurt.

- 180 g rice with vegetables
- 1/3 cup low-fat frozen yogurt with 180 g raspberries

Servings:

- 3 servings of whole-grain products
- 6 fruits
- 5 vegetables
- 3 (+/-) servings of dairy products
- 40 g nuts
- 210 g meat

Third week.

Breakfast: Cornflakes, toast, juice, and milk.
- 30 g cornflakes with 180 g strawberries
- 1 whole-grain toast with 2 tsp. orange jam
- 180 ml apple juice
- 240 ml low-fat milk

Lunch: Grilled chicken with salad, orange.
- 180 g of grilled chicken
- Green salad: 1 cup vegetables
- 1 medium orange

Snack: Yogurt with berries.
- 180 ml low-fat yogurt
- 1/3 cup different berries
- 40 g nuts

Dinner: Cheese sandwich with salad, pineapple, and frozen yogurt
- Sandwich: 2 pieces whole-grain bread with 40 g low-fat cheese and 3 slices tomato
- 150 g pineapple
- ¼ cup frozen yogurt with fruits

Servings:
- 3 servings of whole-grain products
- 4-5 fruits
- 5-6 vegetables
- 4 servings of dairy products
- 40 g nuts
- 180 g meat

Breakfast: corn flakes with a toast and a glass of juice.
- 30 g cornflakes with 180 g of strawberries
- 180 ml apple juice
- 1 whole-grain toast with 2 tsp. blueberry jam
- 230 ml low-fat milk

Lunch: chicken sandwich, and a green salad.
- Small sandwich with chicken breast
- Salad: lettuce, 9 cherry tomatoes. 2 tbsp. low-fat dressing
- 230 ml milk
- 1 medium orange

Snack: fresh yogurt with nuts.
- ¼ cup peanuts
- 180 ml of raspberry yogurt (sugar-free)

Dinner: chicken chop with potatoes, green salad, green beans, cookies, and grapes.
- 180 g chicken chop
- ½ cup green beans
- Green salad with 2 tbsp. olive oil and vinegar

- 2 biscuits
- 1 glass grapes

Daily portions:
- 3 servings of whole grains
- 4 fruits
- 5 vegetables
- 3 serving low-fat dairy products
- 40 g nuts
- 200 g meat

Day 17. Wednesday

Breakfast: Scrambled eggs, toast, pineapple, juice and milk.
- 2 eggs
- 2 whole-grain toast and 4 tsp. orange marmalade
- 180 g pineapple
- 180 ml of cherry juice
- 240 ml of low-fat milk

Lunch: Salad with chicken, whole-grain bread, cabbage salad, milk, strawberries, jelly, and plums.
- ½ salad with chicken
- 1 whole-grain cake
- 1 cup cabbage salad
- 240 ml low-fat milk
- ½ cup strawberries
- 2 small plums

Snack: Yogurt with banana.
- 180 ml low-fat kiwi yogurt
- 1 medium banana

Dinner: Grilled chicken with potatoes, green salad, and frozen yogurt.
- Grilled chicken – 120 g
- 1 cup potatoes
- 1 cup asparagus
- Salad: 1 ½ cup greens and vegetables, 2 tbsp. olive oil and vinegar
- 1 cup low-fat yogurt

Servings:
- 3 servings of the whole-grain products
- 4 (+/-) fruits
- 6 vegetables
- 4 servings of low-fat dairy products
- 240 g meat

Day 18. Thursday

Breakfast: Toast with fruits and a fresh smoothie.
- 2 whole-grain toast with the ½ cup sliced strawberries
- Smoothie: 120 g cherries, ½ banana and 240 ml low-fat milk

Lunch: Sandwich with tuna and cheese, potatoes, cabbage salad, milk and some fruits.

- Sandwich: ½ cup of tuna, 30 g of low-fat cheese and 1 piece of whole-grain bread
- 1 serving of baked potatoes
- 1 serving of cabbage salad
- ½ cup steamed peas and carrots
- 240 ml low-fat milk
- 1 medium banana

Afternoon snack: Fresh carrots, cheese, almond
- 5 small fresh carrots with low-fat cheese
- ¼ cup almond

Dinner: Grilled chicken with vegetables, baked potatoes, spinach, plums.
- Grilled chicken
- ½ cup young vegetables and 4 tomatoes with 2 tbsp. dressing
- ½ cup baked potatoes
- ½ cup spinach
- 2 plumps

Daily servings:
- 3 servings of whole grains
- 4 fruits
- 5-6 vegetables
- 3 servings of dairy products
- 40 g nuts
- 180 g meat

Day 19. Friday

Breakfast: Omelet, raspberries, toast, juice, and milk.
- Omelet: ½ cup milk-egg mixture
- 180 g sliced raspberry
- 1 whole-grain toast with 2 tsp. blueberry jam
- 180 ml apple juice
- 240 ml low-fat milk

Lunch: Sandwich with beef and cheese, potato chips (home-made) with tomatoes, a glass of milk and some fruits.
- Sandwich: 2 pieces of whole-grain bread, 60 g lean meat, 30 g low-fat cheese, ¼ cup of lettuce, 2 slices tomato and mustard (or without it)
- 30 g low-salted potato chips cooked in the oven
- 4 tomatoes
- 230 ml low-fat milk
- 180 g pineapple

Afternoon snack: Peach slices and low-fat yogurt.
- 1 medium sliced peach
- 1 low-fat yogurt

Dinner: Spaghetti with low-fat sauce, green beans, lettuce and frozen yogurt for a dessert.
- Spaghetti with the low-fat sauce: 1 cup sauce and 1 cup spaghetti
- ½ cup green beans
- Green salad: ½ cup lettuce with 2 tbsp. low-fat Italian sauce, without salt
- ½ cup frozen chocolate yogurt

Servings:
- 3 servings of whole-grain bread
- 4 fruits
- 5 vegetables
- 4 (+/-) servings of low-fat dairy products
- 40 g nuts
- 200 g meat

Day 20. Saturday

Breakfast: English muffin with cheese, melon, juice, and milk.
- 1 muffin with raisins and low-fat cheese
- 180 g pineapple
- 180 ml cherry juice
- 240 ml low-fat milk

Lunch: Pork tacos with peach.
- 90 g lean meat for tacos
- 30 g low-fat cheese
- Sliced tomatoes and romaine salad, grated carrots and chopped red cabbage
- 1 medium peach

Snack: Orange, popcorn, cheese.
- 1 medium orange
- 2 cups popcorn
- 1 piece of low-fat cheese

Dinner: Steak, baked potatoes, broccoli, lettuce.
- 120 g beef steak
- 1 baked potato
- ½ cup broccoli
- Salad: 1 ½ of leafy vegetables with 2 tbsp. of French sauce
- 1 piece of whole-grain bread with 1 tsp. of soft margarine
- 180 ml low-fat peach yogurt (sugar-free)

Daily servings:
- 5 servings of whole-grain products
- 4 fruits
- 5 vegetables
- 3 (+/-) servings of dairy products
- 40 g nuts
- 210 g meat

Day 21. Sunday

Breakfast: Omelet with cheese, cookies, milk, and juice.
- Omelet with low-fat cheese
- 180 ml apple juice
- 240 ml low-fat milk
- 2 biscuits

Lunch: Cheese with avocado, cucumber salad, and peaches.
- 2 pieces of whole-grain bread, 20 g low-fat cheese and 2 avocado slices

- ¾ cup cucumber slices and 1 tbsp. low-fat Italian dressing.
- 1 peach

Snack: Yogurt, peanuts, and pineapple.
- 180 ml low-fat strawberry yogurt.
- ¼ cup roasted peanut (without salt)
- 180 g pineapple

Dinner: Grilled chicken with potatoes, vegetables, pudding and some fruits.
- 1 serving of grilled chicken with potatoes, carrots, Brussel sprouts
- ½ cup of chocolate pudding
- 1 medium pear

Servings:
- 2 servings of whole-grain products
- 5 fruits
- 5 (+/-) vegetables
- 3 (+/-) servings of dairy products
- 40 g of nuts
- 240 g of lean meat

The last week.

Breakfast: Cornflakes, pineapple, cherry juice, milk.

- 45 g corn flakes
- 180 g pineapple
- 180 ml cherry juice
- 240 ml low-fat milk

Lunch: Cheese, green salad, fresh vegetables, and orange.

- 2 pieces of whole-grain bread with 30 ml low-fat cheese and 2 slices of tomato
- Salad: 1 cup vegetables with 2 tbsp. of French sauce
- 8 small carrots
- 1 medium apple

Snack: Blueberry smoothie with almonds.

- Smoothie: 240 ml low-fat milk and 180 g blueberries
- 40 g almonds

Dinner: Grilled chicken with rice and tomatoes. Cheese and lettuce.

- 1 serving of grilled chicken
- 1 cup brown rice
- ½ cup tomatoes with 30 g melted low-fat cheese
- Salad: 1 ½ cup vegetables with 2 tbsp. of dressing

Daily servings:

- 3 servings of whole-grain products
- 1 serving nuts
- 5 fruits
- 3 servings dairy products
- 210 g lean meat

Breakfast: Cornflakes, melon, milk, and juice.

- 45 g cornflakes
- 150 g melon
- 180 ml strawberry juice
- 240 ml milk

Lunch: Pita with tuna, salad, and grapes.

- Pita with tuna: ½ whole-grain pita with ½ cup tuna and with 2 slices of tomato
- Salad: 1 cup leafy vegetables with 2 tbsp. of dressing
- 180 g grapes

Snack: Peanuts with apples.

- ¼ cup peanuts
- 2 medium apples

Dinner: Cheeseburger with cabbage salad, and ice-cream.

- Low-fat cheeseburger: 120 g low-fat beef, 30 g low-fat cheese, 2 tomato slices, lettuce and bread for burger
- ½ cabbage salad
- 1 cup broccoli and carrots

- Ice-cream: 30 g strawberries with low-fat frozen yogurt

Daily servings:
- 2 servings of whole-grain products
- 4 fruits
- 5 vegetables
- 3 servings of dairy products
- 40 g nuts
- 210 g meat

Day 24. Wednesday

Breakfast: Bagel with cheese, some fruits, latte, and juice.
- ½ of whole-grain bagel with low-fat cheese
- 180 g strawberries
- 240 ml low-fat milk for latte
- 180 ml grapefruit juice

Lunch: Burrito with cheese and beans, lettuce, and apples.
- 1 burrito with ½ cup beans and 20 g low-fat cheese
- ½ cup corn
- Salad: 1 cup lettuce, tomatoes, and carrots with 1 tbsp. nuts, and 1 tbsp. olive oil
- 2 small plums

Snack: Latte, cookies, fruit salad.
- Coffee Latte
- 2 biscuits
- ½ cup of fruit salad

Dinner: Steak with salad, fruit chips.
- 120 g of steak
- Green salad: 1 ½ cup vegetables with 2 tbsp. olive oil and vinegar
- ½ cup fruit crisps with ½ cup low-fat frozen yogurt

Servings:
- 3 servings of whole-grain products
- 5 fruits
- 5 vegetables
- 5 serving of low-fat dairy products
- 40 g beans
- 120 g meat

Day 25. Thursday

Breakfast: Scrambled eggs, melon, juice, milk.
- Scrambled eggs with 3 slices of tomato
- 180 g melon
- 180 g cherry juice
- 240 ml low-fat milk for latte

Lunch: Spaghetti Bolognese, salad, juice, and berries.
- 150 g spaghetti Bolognese
- Salad: 1 cup fresh vegetables with 2 tbsp. olive oil
- 180 ml apple juice

- 1/3 cup berries

Snack: Tomato soup, orange.

- ¾ cup tomato soup
- 1 medium banana

Dinner: Rice with vegetables, and frozen yogurt.

- 180 g rise with vegetables
- 1/3 cup low-fat frozen yogurt with 180 g blueberries

Servings:

- 3 servings of whole-grain products
- 6 fruits
- 5 vegetables
- 3 (+/-) servings of dairy products
- 40 g nuts
- 210 g meat

Day 26. Friday

Breakfast: Cornflakes, pineapple, milk, and raspberry juice.

- 40 g of corn flakes
- 180 g pineapple
- 180 ml raspberry juice
- 240 ml milk

Lunch: Pita with tuna, salad, and melon.

- Pita with tuna: ½ whole-grain pita with ½ cup tuna and with 2 slices of tomato
- Salad: 1 cup leafy vegetables with 2 tbsp. of dressing
- 180 g melon

Snack: Peanuts with plums

- ¼ cup of peanuts
- 2 plums

Dinner: Cheeseburger with cabbage salad and ice-cream.

- Low-fat cheeseburger: 120 g low-fat beef, 30 g low-fat cheese, 2 tomato slices, lettuce and bread for burger
- ½ cabbage salad
- 1 cup broccoli and carrots
- Ice-cream: 30 g strawberries with low-fat frozen yogurt

Daily servings:

- 2 servings of whole-grain products
- 4 fruits
- 5 vegetables
- 3 servings of dairy products
- 40 g nuts
- 210 g meat

Day 27. Saturday

Breakfast: Oatmeal, banana, toast, grapefruit, and milk

- ½ cup oatmeal with small pieces of banana
- 1 whole-grain toast with 2 tsp. strawberry jam

- 180 g grapefruit
- 240 ml low-fat milk

Lunch: Soup, cheese, yogurt, and apples
- 1 cup vegetable soup
- 30 g low-fat cheese
- 180 ml low-fat yogurt
- 2 small oranges

Snack: Cheese and berries.
- 40 g nuts
- 1/3 cup different fresh berries

Dinner: Pork chop with baked potatoes, green beans, carrot salad, walnuts, and milk.
- 120 g fried pork chop
- ½ cup baked potatoes
- 1 cup green beans
- ½ cup carrot salad with ¼ cup of nuts
- 100 ml red wine

Daily servings:
- 3 portions of whole-grain products
- 4 fruits
- 7 vegetables
- 4 (+/-) servings of dairy products
- 1 serving of nuts
- 120 g meat
- 1 glass of wine

Day 28. Sunday

Breakfast: Cornflakes with pieces of banana, cherry juice, and latte.
- 45 g cornflakes with small pieces of banana
- 180 ml cherry juice
- 240 ml low-fat milk for latte

Lunch: Green salad with mushrooms, melon, and juice.
- 1 cup leafy vegetables for the green salad with 2 tbsp. of French sauce
- ½ cup grilled mushrooms
- 180 g melon
- 150 ml apple juice

Snack: Low-fat yogurt with nuts and some fruits
- 180 ml low-fat yogurt with pieces of fruits
- 40 g nuts

Dinner: Spaghetti Bolognese with red wine, beans, and frozen yogurt
- 200 g spaghetti
- 150 ml red wine
- 1/3 cup beans
- ¼ cup chocolate frozen yogurt

Daily servings:
- 3 servings of whole-grain products
- 3 servings of low-fat dairy products

- 4 fruits
- 5-6 vegetables

4. Breakfast recipes

Poached eggs on toast with avocado slices.

Ingredients:

- 2 eggs
- 2 slices of whole-grain bread
- 6 slices of avocado
- 2 tbsp. Parmesan cheese
- Ground pepper
- Basil (or any other fresh herbs) for topping

Instructions:

1. Crack 2 eggs into the boiling water and wait for 2 minutes.
2. Then chop avocado and remove the stone.
3. With the help of knife or fork smash the avocado slices on the toasts.
4. Sprinkle everything with the Parmesan cheese and pepper.
5. Use basil for topping.

Notes

Scrambled eggs with spinach.

Ingredients:

- 2 eggs
- ½ tsp. fresh basil
- ½ tsp. pepper
- ¼ cup low-fat cheese
- 1 big chopped spinach
- 1 medium chopped tomato

Instructions:

1. In medium bowl mix eggs, pepper, and basil until frothy.
2. Pour into the prepared frying pan. Add spinach and tomato.
3. Cook for 5 minutes.
4. When everything is ready sprinkle with cheese and ground pepper.

Notes

Oatmeal with blueberries and milk.

Ingredients:

- ½ cup oatmeal
- ½ cup blueberries
- 1 tbsp. sunflower seeds
- 100 ml low-fat milk

Instructions:

1. Take a small saucepan and bring the milk to a boil.
2. Add oatmeal and cook for 2-3 minutes more.
3. When the oatmeal is ready, add sunflower seeds and blueberries.
4. Pour everything with milk.

Notes

Scrambled eggs with beans, tomatoes, and pesto.

Ingredients:

- 3 eggs
- 3 tsp olive oil
- ¼ tsp. salt
- ¼ tsp. pepper
- ½ cup grape tomatoes
- ½ cup low-sodium canned white beans
- 2 slices whole-grain bread

Instructions:

1. In a medium bowl mix eggs with salt and pepper.
2. Then place eggs on the frying pan. Add olive oil. Fry them 5 minutes.
3. Prepare tomatoes with beans. Take another frying pan and cook them with olive oil for 5 minutes.
4. Make toasts.
5. Serve eggs with the tomato, beans and toasts.

Notes

Yogurt with grapes and granola.

Ingredients:
- 1 cup low-fat yogurt
- ¼ cup red and green grapes
- ½ cup granola

Instructions:
1. In a bowl mix one cup low-fat yogurt and with granola.
2. Then divide it between 2 glasses.
3. Use grapes for topping.

Notes

Morning sunshine smoothie.

Ingredients:

- 200 ml carrot juice
- 80 g pineapple
- ½ banana
- Small piece of ginger
- 10 g cashew nuts

Instructions:

1. Prepare all ingredients that you need.
2. In a blender mix carrot juice, pineapple, banana, ginger and nuts in your blender until smooth.
3. Pour everything into the glasses.
4. Enjoy.

Notes

Low-fat yogurt with fruits and nuts.

Ingredients:

- 180 ml low-fat yogurt
- ¼ cup berries
- ½ sliced banana
- 1 tbsp. sunflower seeds
- 20 g of nuts

Instructions:

1. Mix the nuts with sunflower seeds.
2. Then slice banana.
3. In a bowl mix sliced banana with berries.
4. Add yogurt and pour everything into the glasses.
5. Enjoy.

Notes

Home-made muesli with berries.

Ingredients:

- ½ cup oats
- ½ tsp. sunflower seeds
- ½ tsp. raisins
- ¼ cup dried cranberries
- ¼ cup blueberries
- 100 ml low-fat milk
- 20 g nuts

Instructions:

1. Take a medium bowl. Mix sunflower seeds, raisins, dried cranberries and blueberries with the oats.
2. Divide it between the small bowls.
3. Pour over the low-fat milk.
4. Top with blueberries.

Notes

Tropical breakfast smoothie.

Ingredients:

- ½ banana chopped
- ½ mango chopped
- 180 ml orange juice
- Ice cubes (optional)

Instructions:

1. Chop banana and mango.
2. Put chopped banana and mango in the blender and mix them until smooth.
3. Add orange juice and mix again (for 2 minutes more)
4. Then pour everything into the glasses
5. Enjoy.

<table>
<tr><td>Notes</td></tr>
<tr><td>

</td></tr>
</table>

5. Appetizers and snacks

Tomato basil bruschetta.

Ingredients:

- ½ of whole-grain baguette
- 2 tbsp. chopped basil
- 1 tbsp. chopped parsley
- 1 clove of garlic
- 2 chopped tomatoes
- 1 tsp. olive oil
- 1 tsp. balsamic vinegar
- ½ tsp. pepper

Instructions:

1. Slice baguette.
2. Chop basil, parsley, and tomatoes.
3. Preheat the oven for 2-3 minutes.
4. Put baguette slices into the oven (400F). And wait until they become brown.
5. In a medium bowl mix chopped basil, parsley, tomatoes with garlic, pepper and olive oil.
6. Then pour the mixture over the slices.
7. Enjoy.

Notes

Grilled pineapple with cinnamon.

Ingredients:

- 1 tbsp. honey
- ½ tbsp. olive oil
- 1 tbsp. lemon juice
- 1 tsp. cinnamon
- ½ pineapple
- ½ tbsp. grated lime

Instructions:

1. Prepare grill with cooking spray. And then preheat it to high.
2. In a medium bowl mix honey with cinnamon, olive oil, juice.
3. Clear the pineapple.
4. Cut pineapple.
5. Pour out the marinade on the pineapple slices.
6. Grill them until golden color. 5 minutes for each side.
7. Enjoy.

Notes

Creamy apple cinnamon smoothie.

Ingredients:

- ½ banana
- ½ apple
- 2 tbsp. oats
- 1 tbsp. almond butter
- 100 ml almond milk
- ¼ tsp. cinnamon

Instructions:

1. In the blender mix banana, apple with almond butter and milk. Blend them until creamy.
2. Divide it between the glasses (or cups)
3. Use granola for topping.

Notes

Baked zucchini chips.

Ingredients:

- 1 medium zucchini
- ¼ cup whole-grain breadcrumbs
- ¼ cup low-fat cheese
- ¼ tsp. pepper
- Garlic
- 3 tbsp. low-fat milk

Instructions:

1. Preheat oven to 220 degrees.
2. In a bowl mix breadcrumbs with pepper, cheese, and garlic.
3. Make zucchini slices.
4. Then prepare baking sheet.
5. Dip zucchini slices into milk and then into the breadcrumbs (from both sides).
6. Place zucchini slices on baking sheet and bake them until golden color (for 1,5-2 hours)

Notes

Toast with creamy cheese, berries, and basil.

Ingredients:

- 1 slice whole-grain bread
- 20 g low-fat creamy cheese
- 30 g berries
- basil

Instructions:

1. Make a toast.
2. Add creamy cheese.
3. Use berries and basil for topping.

<table>
<tr><td>Notes</td></tr>
</table>

The mix of low-fat yogurt, nuts, and fresh fruits.

Ingredients:

- 180 ml low-fat yogurt
- 30 g nuts
- ½ banana
- ¼ cup strawberries

Instructions:

1. In a bowl mix banana, strawberries, and nuts.
2. Add yogurt and mix again.
3. Divide everything between the glasses.
4. Enjoy.

Notes

Homemade sweet potato chips.

Ingredients:
- 3 potatoes
- 2 tbsp. olive oil
- ½ tsp. pepper

Instructions:
1. Preheat the oven to 400 degrees.
2. Clean potatoes and slice them.
3. Pour all slices with olive oil and add pepper.
4. Place slices on the baking sheet and cook them in the oven for 20-25 minutes.
5. When everything is ready, sprinkle with salt.

Notes

Fresh tomato crostini.

Ingredients:
- 2 chopped tomatoes
- ¼ cup fresh basil
- 2 tsp. olive oil
- ½ of garlic
- ½ spoon pepper
- ¼ of Italian bread

Instructions:
1. Make toasts.
2. Chop tomatoes.
3. In a medium bowl mix chopped tomatoes, olive oil, basil, and pepper. Leave this mixture for 2 hours.
4. Add mixture to the toasts and enjoy your meal.

Notes

Crispy potato skins.

- 2 potatoes
- 1 tbsp. rosemary
- 1/8 tsp. pepper
- Cooking spray

Instructions:

1. Preheat the oven to 400 degrees.
2. Clean potatoes and bake them until the skins are crisp (for 60-75 minutes)
3. Take a cooking spray and spray each potato.
4. Press the rosemary and pepper. And add it to the potatoes.
5. Serve on a plate.

Notes

Fresh tomato crostini.

Ingredients:
- 4 chopped tomatoes
- ¼ cup fresh basil
- 2 tsp olive oil
- 1 tsp pepper
- 1 clove garlic (minced)
- 4 slices of whole-grain bread

Instructions:
1. Chop all tomatoes.
2. Mince garlic.
3. In a bowl combine chopped tomatoes with fresh basil, olive oil, pepper, and minced garlic.
4. Wait until the tomato mixture is ready.
5. Make toasts.
6. Smear the mixture on toasts.\

<table>
<tr><td>Notes</td></tr>
</table>

6. Soups, salads, and sandwiches

Fresh citrus salad.

Ingredients:

- 1 orange
- 1 grapefruit
- 2 tbsp. orange juice
- 1 tbsp. olive oil
- 2 cups spring greens
- 2 tbsp. pine nuts
- 1 tbsp. chopped mint

Instructions:

1. Make orange and grapefruit slices.
2. In a small bowl make a mixture of olive oil and orange juice.
3. In another bowl mix spring greens and pine nuts with the first mixture.
4. Then add orange and grapefruit slices.
5. Chop mint.
6. Divide everything between the plates.
7. Serve topped with chopped mint.

Notes

Potato salad.

Ingredients:
- 2 boiled potatoes
- ½ onion
- ½ carrot
- 2 tbsp. olive oil
- ½ tsp. pepper
- 1 tsp. wine vinegar
- ¼ cup low-fat mayonnaise

Instructions:
1. Cut all vegetables.
2. Take olive oil, pepper, wine vinegar and low-fat mayonnaise. Mix them in the medium bowl to make a sauce.
3. Add this sauce to the vegetables. Mix it. And your salad is ready.
4. Divide it between the plates.

Notes

Grilled chicken salad with olives and oranges.

Ingredients:

- 2 tbsp. wine vinegar.
- 1 garlic clove
- 1 tbsp. olive oil
- 1 tbsp. chopped onion
- ½ spoon pepper
- 300 g chicken

Instructions:

1. Chop onion.
2. For making the dressing combine the vinegar, garlic, chopped onion, olive oil, and pepper in a medium bowl.
3. Rub the meat with garlic.
4. Grill chicken until brown color (for 30 minutes)
5. Then make chicken slices and pour sauce on them.
6. Serve immediately.

Notes

Easy vegetable soup.

Ingredients:

- 2 tsp. olive oil
- 12 chopped mushrooms
- 1 medium onion
- 2 large carrots
- 5 cloves garlic
- 6 cups water
- 5 fresh parsley springs
- 2 celery stalks
- 3 fresh thyme springs
- 1 bay leaf
- 1/8 tsp. salt

Instructions:

1. Chop all mushrooms.
2. In a saucepan heat 2 tsp. olive oil, add chopped mushrooms and wait (4-5 minutes) until brown color.
3. Add plus 1 tsp. olive oil, onion, celery, carrots and garlic to the mushrooms.
4. Wait until the vegetables become browner.
5. Then add the water, bay leaf, thyme, parsley, and salt.
6. Bring it to the boil and simmer for 20 minutes.
7. Remove from the heat and let it cool.
8. Take a blender and mix it.
9. Pour into the bowls.
10. Serve immediately.

Notes

Easy carrot soup.

- 10 sliced carrots
- ½ tbsp. sugar
- 2 cups water
- ¼ tsp. ground pepper
- ¼ tsp. nutmeg
- 3 tbsp. flour
- 3 cups fat-free milk
- 2 tbsp. fresh chopped parsley

1. Slice all carrots.
2. In the big pot put sliced carrots, sugar, and water. Heat them.
3. Then simmer it for 20 minutes.
4. In another saucepan mix flour, pepper, fat-free milk, and nutmeg. Cook the sauce 10-15 minutes.
5. In the blender mix cooked carrots and sauce until smooth. Add some water.
6. Pour ready soup into the bowls.
7. Use parsley for topping.
8. Enjoy.

Notes

Fresh tuna sandwiches.

Ingredients:
- 2 canes unsalted tuna
- ½ cup diced celery
- 1 tsp. lemon juice
- ¼ cup fat-free mayonnaise
- 4 lettuce leaves
- 8 slices of the whole-grain bread

Instructions:
1. In a bowl mix tuna with celery, lemon juice, and mayonnaise.
2. Slice bread.
3. Put one lettuce leaf on a slice of bread. Add tuna mixture. Then add another slice of bread again.
4. Enjoy.

Notes

Grilled mushrooms burgers.

Ingredients:

- 4 large cups of mushrooms.
- 1/3 cup vinegar
- ½ cup water
- 1 tbsp. sugar
- ½ garlic clove
- ¼ tsp. pepper
- 1 tbsp. olive oil
- 4 toasts
- 4 slices tomato
- 4 slices onion

Instructions:

1. Slice tomato and onion.
2. In a medium bowl mix vinegar, water, sugar, garlic, olive oil and cayenne pepper for making the sauce.
3. Pour this sauce over mushrooms. Leave them for 1 hour.
4. Prepare grill for the medium heat.
5. Grill mushrooms about 5-6 minutes, using a marinade.
6. Put each mushroom on a bun.
7. Serve topped with a tomato slice, onion slice and half of the lettuce leaf.

<table>
<tr><td>Notes</td></tr>
</table>

Tasty spiced Asian salad.

Ingredients:

- 2 cups chopped melon (watermelon)
- ½ cup low-fat yogurt
- ¼ tsp. mace
- 1/8 tsp. clove
- 1/8 tsp. cinnamon
- 3 tbsp. orange juice

Instructions:

1. Chop melon (or watermelon).
2. Take a large bowl and mix low-fat yogurt, mace, clove, cinnamon with orange juice.
3. Add chopped melon. And mix it.
4. Divide salad between the plates.
5. Enjoy.

Notes

English cucumber salad.

Ingredients:

- 2 cucumbers
- ½ tsp. pepper
- 1 tbsp. chopped fresh rosemary
- 2 tbsp. balsamic vinegar
- 2 tbsp. olive oil
- 1 tbsp. mustard

Instructions:

1. Slice cucumbers.
2. Chop rosemary.
3. In a bowl mix olive oil, balsamic vinegar, mustard, and pepper.
4. Add dressing to the salad.
5. Divide it between the plates.
6. Enjoy your meal.

Notes

Cherry tomato salad.

Ingredients:

- 2 tbsp. vinegar
- 1 tbsp. olive oil
- ¼ tsp. salt
- 1/8 tsp. pepper
- 1 ½ cups yellow pear tomatoes
- 1 ½ cups orange cherry tomatoes
- 1 ½ cup red cherry tomatoes
- 4 large leaves (basil)

Instructions:

1. In a bowl mix vinegar, olive oil, pepper and salt for making the dressing.
2. Chop all tomatoes, cut basil leaves.
3. Mix chopped tomatoes with cut basil leaves.
4. Add dressing.
5. Serve immediately.

Notes

Cucumber salad with pineapple.

Ingredients:
- 2 tbsp. sugar
- 2 tbsp. vinegar
- 1 tbsp. water
- ½ cup pineapple
- 1 medium cucumber
- ½ carrot
- ¼ cup sliced onion
- 2 cups salad greens
- ½ tbsp. sesame seeds

Instructions:
1. In a small saucepan boil sugar, vinegar, and water for 3 minutes. Wait until cool.
2. Then add pineapple. Wait for 1 hour.
3. Add chopped cucumbers, carrots and red onions to this mixture.
4. Divide it between the plates.
5. For the topping use salad greens.

Notes

7.Entrees

Grilled beef with basil.

Ingredients:

- 1 tsp. fresh lemon juice
- 1/5 cup olive oil
- ¼ tsp. pepper
- 1 ½ cups of basil leaves
- 2 garlic cloves
- ½ tsp. salt
- 200 g of steak
- 80 g white beans
- ½ cup grape tomatoes
- 1 tbsp. chopped red onion

Instructions:

1. In a bowl combine lemon juice, olive oil, pepper, basil leaves for making the sauce.
2. Grill meat for 5-6 minutes.
3. Pour sauce over the meat.
4. Serve topped with white beans.
5. Enjoy.

Notes

Roast beef with fresh herbs.

Ingredients:

- 200 g meat
- ½ cup chopped mint, rosemary, and tarragon.
- ½ tsp. pepper
- 2 tbsp. olive oil
- 1 cup fresh basil leaves

Instructions:

1. Preheat your oven to 180 C.
2. Heat 1 tsp. olive oil.
3. Grill meat until brown color for 25-30 minutes.
4. In a bowl make a sauce from basil, olive oil, and salt.
5. Chop mint, rosemary, and tarragon.
6. Slice meat and add chopped herbs to basil oil.

Notes

Grilled salmon with mushrooms.

Ingredients:
- 1 tbsp. olive oil
- 1 tbsp. fresh ginger
- 1 tbsp. wine vinegar
- 250 g salmon
- 50 g mushrooms

Instructions:
1. In a bowl combine olive oil, fresh ginger, and wine vinegar.
2. Add the salmon to the mixture.
3. Preheat grill to medium.
4. Grill salmon with mushrooms for 5 minutes.
5. Enjoy.

Notes

Crusted chicken with honey.

Ingredients:

- 6 saltine crackers
- 1 tsp. paprika
- 250 g chicken
- 3 tsp. honey

Instructions:

1. Crush the crackers and put them in the bowl. Add paprika. And mix it.
2. Mix chicken with honey and ad cracker mixture.
3. Preheat the oven to 180 C.
4. Prepare the baking dish.
5. Then cook chicken for 20-30 minutes.
6. Serve immediately.

Notes

Roasted salmon with basil.

Ingredients:
- 250 g salmon
- 2 tsp. olive oil
- 1 tbsp. chopped chives
- 1 tbsp. basil

Instructions:
1. Rub salmon with 2 tsp. olive oil.
2. Preheat the oven to 200 C.
3. Place salmon on the baking sheet and cook it for 15-20 minutes.
4. Chop chives.
5. Top ready salmon with chopped chives and basil.

<table>
<tr><td>Notes</td></tr>
</table>

Pasta with spinach and raisins.

Ingredients:

- 200 g pasta
- 2 tbsp. olive oil
- 1 garlic clove
- ¼ cup raisins
- 1 cup fresh spinach
- 2 tbsp. Parmesan cheese

Instructions:

1. Fill a pot full with water, add the pasta and cook it for 12-15 minutes (or according to the package directions). Then drain the pasta.
2. In a large skillet heat the olive oil with garlic. Add the raisins and spinach.
3. Cook it about 3 minutes more (but don't overcook it)
4. Add it to the cooked pasta.
5. Divide it between the plates.
6. Top pasta with sauce and cheese.

Notes

Pasta with pumpkin sauce.

Ingredients:

- 200 g pasta
- 2 tsp. olive oil
- ½ onion chopped
- ½ clove garlic
- 5 mushrooms
- ½ cup vegetables
- 50 g pumpkin
- 1/5 ground pepper
- ¼ tsp. sage
- 2 tbsp. Parmesan cheese
- 1 tsp. parsley

Instructions:

1. In a medium saucepan boil pasta for 15 minutes (or according to the directions)
2. Take a medium skillet and fry mushrooms, onion, and garlic with olive oil for 7 minutes.
3. Then add vegetables, pumpkin, sage, and salt. And cook 8 minutes more.
4. Add sauce to the pasta.
5. Sprinkle with cheese and parsley.

<table>
<tr><td>Notes</td></tr>
</table>

Pasta with grilled chicken and mushrooms.

- 180 g chicken
- 1 tbsp. olive oil
- ¼ cup chopped onion
- 20 g sliced mushrooms
- ½ cup of cooked beans
- 1 tbsp. garlic
- 1/5 cup chopped fresh basil
- 200 g pasta
- 2 tbsp. Parmesan cheese
- ½ tsp. ground black pepper

Instructions:

1. Grill chicken breast until brown color.
2. Then slice chicken into strips.
3. Chop onions and slice mushrooms. Fry them together for 7 minutes more.
4. Then add garlic, beans, basil and chicken strips.
5. Take a saucepan and cook pasta for 10 minutes.
6. To the cooked pasta add chicken mixture.
7. Divide everything between the plates.
8. Sprinkle with Parmesan cheese.

Notes

Broccoli with garlic and rigatoni.

Ingredients:

- 200 g rigatoni noodles
- 1 cup broccoli
- 1 tbsp. Parmesan cheese
- 1 tsp. olive oil
- 1 tsp. minced garlic
- ½ tsp. pepper

Instructions:

1. Take a saucepan to boil rigatoni noodles (10-15 minutes)
2. Take another saucepan and put broccoli into the hot water and steam it about 10 minutes.
3. When everything is ready, combine pasta with broccoli.
4. Mince garlic.
5. Sprinkle with Parmesan cheese, olive oil, and minced garlic.

Notes

Fried rice with vegetables.

Ingredients:

- 1 cup cooked rice
- 1 tbsp. peanut oil
- 1 chopped onion
- 1 carrot
- ¼ cup chopped green pepper
- 1 egg
- 1 tbsp. sesame oil
- 2 tbsp. chopped parsley

Instructions:

1. Take a small saucepan and bring the water to the boil.
2. Then to the hot water add rice and simmer it for 20 minutes.
3. Heat the peanut oil and add cooked rice.
4. Chop onions and parsley.
5. Take a large skillet, preheat it and add chopped onions, carrots, pepper. Fry them about 5 minutes.
6. Mix vegetables with rice. Break the egg into the mixture. And cook it.
7. When everything is ready, sprinkle with the sesame oil and chopped parsley.

<table><tr><td>Notes</td></tr><tr><td>

</td></tr></table>

8.Desserts

Creamy fruit dessert.

Ingredients:

- 100 g low-fat cream cheese
- ¼ cup low-fat yogurt
- 1 tsp. sugar
- ¼ tsp. vanilla
- 10 orange slices
- 10 peaches slices
- 10 pineapple slices
- 2 tbsp. coconut

Instructions:

1. In a bowl combine vanilla, sugar, cream cheese and yogurt. Using a mixer, beat all ingredients until smooth.
2. Slice all fruits.
3. In the other bowl combine oranges, pineapple, and peaches.
4. Mix sliced fruits with sauce.
5. Enjoy your meal.

Notes

Grapes and walnuts in lemon sauce.

Ingredients:

- ½ cup low-fat sour cream
- 1 tbsp. sugar
- ½ tsp. lemon zest
- ½ tsp. lemon juice
- 1 cup green grapes
- 1 cup red grapes
- 3 tbsp. chopped walnuts

Instructions:

1. In a small bowl combine sour cream, powdered sugar, lemon zest and lemon juice. Mix them. Cover and wait for 2-3 hours.
2. Divide grapes among dessert glasses.
3. Then add lemon topping to the grapes.
4. Chop nuts.
5. Sprinkle with chopped walnuts.

Notes

Sliced orange with citrus syrup.

Ingredients:

- 3 oranges
- 1 cup fresh orange juice
- 2 tbsp. honey
- 2 tbsp. orange liqueur
- 3 mint springs

Instructions:

1. Slice oranges.
2. In a bowl mix orange juice, honey, and orange liqueur to make a sauce.
3. Pour the sauce over the orange slices.
4. Sprinkle with mint springs.

Notes

Rainbow ice pops.

Ingredients:

- 1 ½ cup watermelon, strawberries, and raspberries.
- ½ cup blueberries
- 2 cups fresh apple juice
- 5 cups
- 5 sticks

Instructions:

1. In a medium bowl mix all fruits with apple juice. Then divide them into the cups.
2. Put cups in the fridge. Wait 1 hour.
3. Insert craft sticks into each pop.

Notes

Strawberries with low-fat cream.

Ingredients:

- 1 ½ cup low-fat sour cream
- 2 tbsp. brown sugar
- 2 tbsp. amaretto liqueur
- 250 g fresh strawberries

Instructions:

1. In a medium bowl mix low-fat sour cream with sugar and liqueur.
2. Chop strawberries.
3. Combine the sour cream mixture with chopped strawberries.
4. Serve topped with whole strawberries.

Notes

Morning orange dream.

Ingredients:

- 1 ½ cups orange juice
- 1 cup soy milk
- 1/3 cup soft tofu
- 1 tbsp. honey
- 1 tsp. orange zest
- ¼ tsp. vanilla
- 4 ice cubes
- Orange slices

Instructions:

1. Make orange slices.
2. Take a blender and mix orange juice with soy milk, tofu, orange zest, vanilla, ice cubes and honey. Blend all ingredients until smooth.
3. Pour into glasses and add orange slices.
4. Enjoy it.

<table>
<tr><td>Notes</td></tr>
</table>

Fresh poached pears.

Ingredients:

- 1 cup orange juice
- ¼ cup apple juice
- 4 pears
- 1 tsp. cinnamon
- 1 tsp. nutmeg
- ½ cup blueberries
- 2 tbsp. orange zest

Instructions:

1. In a small saucepan combine juices with cinnamon and nutmeg. Mix them.
2. Peel pears and slice them. Then add sliced pears into the mixture.
3. Simmer it for 20 minutes, but don't boil.
4. Wait until it cool.
5. Serve topped with orange zest.
6. Enjoy.

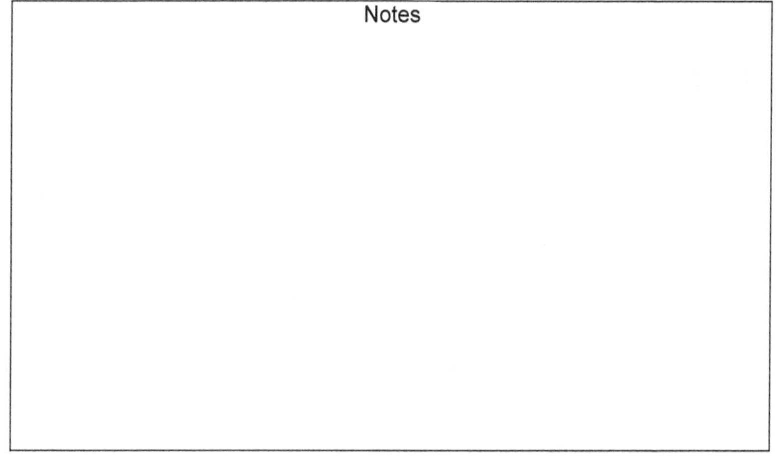

Notes

Poached peaches with vanilla.

- 1 cup water
- 2 tbsp. sugar
- 2 tbsp. vanilla
- 3 peaches
- Mint leaves

Instructions:

1. In a medium nonaluminum saucepan mix vanilla, sugar with water. Boil until the sugar dissolves.
2. Add chopped peaches and wait 7 minutes more.
3. When everything is ready, use mint leaves for topping.
4. Serve it.

<table><tr><td>Notes</td></tr><tr><td>

</td></tr></table>

Strawberry sorbet with balsamic.

Ingredients:

- 1/3 cup balsamic vinegar
- 3 cups strawberries
- 1 tbsp. honey

Instructions:

1. In a small saucepan heat balsamic vinegar and cook it for 5 minutes. And let it cool.
2. Blend strawberries until smooth.
3. Mix the balsamic with honey and puree. Add strawberry mixture.
4. Freeze this mixture and pour it into the ice-cream maker.
5. Wait for 2-3 hours.
6. Enjoy.

<table>
<tr><td>Notes</td></tr>
</table>

Watermelon smoothie with cranberry juice.

Ingredients:
- 3 cups watermelon
- 200 ml cranberry juice
- ¼ cup lime juice
- 6 lime slices

Instructions:
1. Take a blender and blend watermelon until smooth.
2. Then combine it with juices.
3. Pour into the glasses.
4. Garnish with a slice of lime.

Notes

Conclusion

The DASH diet gives you a great chance to have a second look at your eating habits. It shows you what is good for your health and which products are more beneficial for your body. It also proves you that diet could and should be healthy, without requiring from you to stay hungry all the time. But it requires you to reduce the intake of salt, fast food, sugary drinks and unhealthy snacks. At the same time, this diet is rich in fruits, vegetables, low-fat dairy products, protein and whole grains.

This kind of the diet breaks all stereotypes about usual so-called diet. It is a smart dietary program which helps you to control what and how much you eat during the day. It focuses on the balance between healthy food and sport. That is why it allows you not only to solve your health problems but to make your body fitter. It's a great guide for those who want to lose their extra weight without making any stress for their body. Because it includes as much healthy food as you need for losing weight.

Moreover, one of the biggest benefits of this diet is to lower the risk of such diseases as cancer, heart diseases, heart failure or stroke. Following many dietary standards for health, it also reduces the risk of developing diabetes. And works greatly against high blood pressure.

Following its dietary program as well as all dietary recommendations gives everyone a possibility to feel better very soon. The DASH diet is a flexible and balanced eating plan which has everything that your body needs. That means that you can eat all kinds of foods, it's just very important to restrict the calories and to choose the healthier meals. Going on this diet and doing more sports will just bring you to the dreamed result faster.

Author's Afterthoughts

Thanks ever so much to each of my cherished readers for investing the time read this book!

I know you could have picked from many other books but you chose this one. So a big thanks for downloading this book and reading all way to the end.

If you enjoyed this book or received value from it, I'd like to ask you for a favor. Please take a few minutes to post an honest and heartfelt review on Amazon.com Your support does make a difference and to benefit other people.

Thank You!